Low Carb Food Content List

With Carbohydrate Nutritional Information

What to Enjoy & What to Avoid

Tips on Low Carb Shopping - Eating Out - & More

HR Research Alliance

Table of Contents

What Are Low Carb Diets 4

Benefits of a Low Carb Lifestyle 5

Low Carb Foods to Enjoy 7

Foods to Consider Limiting or Avoid All Together 12

Importance of Meal Planning 18

Managing Sugar Cravings 20

Grocery Shopping Tips for Low-Carb Eating 26

Easy 7 Day Sample Low-Carb Meal Plans 31

List of 50 Fruits With Approximate Carbohydrate Content per 100 grams/3.5 oz/1/2 Cup: 39

List of 50 Vegetables Along with Approximate Carbohydrate Content Per 100 grams/3.5 oz/1/2 Cup: 42

List of 10 Dairy Options Low in Carbs, With Carbohydrate Content Per 100 grams/3.5 oz/1/2 Cups: 45

List of 30 High-Carb Foods with Approximate Carbohydrate Content per 100 grams/3.5 oz/1/2 Cups: 46

What Are Low Carb Diets

A low carbohydrate (low carb) diet focuses on reducing the intake of carbohydrates and increasing the consumption of proteins and fats to use as fuel sources. Carbohydrates are primarily found in sugary foods, pasta's, beverages, and bread's. A low carb diet emphasizes foods such as meat's, fish, eggs, vegetables, fruits, nuts, and seeds.

Benefits of a Low Carb Lifestyle

Weight Loss: Reducing carbs can help people lose weight by lowering insulin levels, which causes the body to burn stored fat for energy.

Improved Blood Sugar Control: A low carb diet can stabilize blood sugar levels, which is beneficial for people with diabetes or insulin resistance.

Better Heart Health: Lowering carb intake can improve heart health by increasing HDL (good) cholesterol and decreasing triglycerides.

Reduced Hunger and Cravings: High-protein and high-fat foods can promote satiety and reduce overall hunger, making it easier to stick to a low carb diet.

Enhanced Mental Clarity and Energy Levels: Many people report increased mental clarity and steady energy levels throughout the day when following a low carb diet.

**Brief Overview of Carbohydrate Types and Their Impact on Health
Simple (sugars) Carbohydrates:**

These are sugars that provide quick energy but can cause spikes in blood sugar levels. Found in processed sweets, sodas, and many other types of processed foods. These should be limited on a low carb diet.

Complex Carbohydrates: These are found in foods like grains, legumes, and starchy vegetables. They provide more sustained energy but can still impact blood sugar levels.

Fiber: A type of carbohydrate that the body cannot digest. Found in vegetables, fruits, nuts, and seeds, fiber is crucial for digestive health and does not spike blood sugar.

A low carb diet encourages the consumption of nutrient-dense, whole foods while minimizing the intake of processed and sugary foods. This dietary approach can lead to numerous health benefits and an overall improved quality of life.

Low Carb Foods to Enjoy

Low Carb Vegetables
Leafy Greens: Spinach, kale, Swiss chard, and other leafy greens are low in carbs and high in vitamins, minerals, and fiber.
Cruciferous Vegetables: Broccoli, cauliflower, Brussels sprouts, and cabbage are nutrient-dense and low in carbs.
Other Low Carb Veggies: Zucchini, bell peppers, asparagus, and mushrooms are excellent choices for a low carb dieter.

Protein Sources

Meat: Beef, pork, lamb, and all other meats are carb-free and high in protein and essential nutrients. Making them great choices for a low carb dieter.

Poultry: Chicken, turkey, and other birds provide high-quality protein without the carbs. Making them excellent choices for low carb diets.

Fish and Seafood: Salmon, tuna, mackerel, Oyster, shrimp, and other fish and seafood are rich in omega-3 fatty acids and low in carbs.

Eggs: A versatile and low carb source of protein and healthy fats. Eggs are a top choice for people on low carb diet.

Healthy Fats

Avocado: Low in carbs and high in healthy monounsaturated fats, fiber, and potassium.

Olive Oil: A heart-healthy fat that is low in carbs and rich in antioxidants.

Coconut Oil: Provides medium-chain triglycerides (MCTs) that can be easily used for energy. Low in carbs, & great for cooking with.
Butter and Ghee: Good sources of healthy fats when consumed in moderation.

Dairy Products

Cheese: Most cheeses are low in carbs and provide protein and calcium.
Greek Yogurt: Lower in carbs compared to regular yogurt and high in protein. Great choice for mixing up delicious low carb smoothies.
Heavy Cream: Low in carbs and can be used to add richness to various dishes.

Nuts and Seeds

Almonds: Low in carbs, high in healthy fats, protein, and fiber. Almond butter can also be an excellent choice for low carb dieters.
Walnuts: Rich in omega-3 fatty acids and low in carbs.

Chia Seeds: High in fiber and low in digestible carbs, perfect for adding to smoothies or yogurt.
Flaxseeds: Provide fiber and omega-3 fatty acids with minimal carbs.

Berries

Strawberries: Lower in carbs compared to other fruits and high in vitamin C and antioxidants.
Raspberries: High in fiber and relatively low in carbs.
Blackberries: Another good low carb berry option, rich in vitamins and minerals. Berries taste great mixed in low carb smoothie recipes.

Beverages

Water: Of course water is the absolute best choice for hydration, with zero carbs. Who doesn't love water...
Herbal Tea's: Carb free and can provide various health benefits depending on the type.

Black Coffee: Plain coffee has no carbs and can be enjoyed in moderation.

Low Carb Snacks
Vegetable Sticks with Dip: Celery, cucumber, and bell peppers with guacamole or a low carb dip.
Cheese Sticks: Convenient and low in carbs, perfect for on-the-go snacking.
Nuts and Seeds: Portable and satisfying, just be mindful of portion sizes due to calorie density.
Boiled Eggs: A quick and easy high-protein snack.

Incorporating these foods into your diet can help you maintain a low carb lifestyle while ensuring you get the necessary nutrients for optimal health. Eating low carb does not have to be bland or boring. There are many low carb food choices that taste excellent as nature intended them to.

Foods to Consider Limiting or Avoid All Together

When following a low carb diet, it's important to be mindful of certain foods that are higher in carbohydrates. Limiting or avoiding these foods can help you stay within your carb limits and achieve your dietary goals, whatever they may be per each individual. These foods may possibly be of concern to you if you are following a low carb diet.

Grains and Starches

Bread: Including white, whole grain, and other types of bread, are higher in carbs and might want to be limited or avoided by one following a low carb diet.

Pasta: Typical pasta made from wheat is high in carbs. When possible opt for low carb alternatives like zucchini noodles or shirataki noodles.

Rice: Both white and brown rice are high in carbs. Cauliflower rice is a low carb alternative that also tastes delicious when prepared properly.

Cereal: Most breakfast cereals, even those labeled as healthy, are high in carbs and sugars. These are also processed foods which should be limited or avoided by most people on low carb diets.

Sugary Foods and Beverages

Sweets and Candy: High in sugar and carbs, these should be avoided on a low carb diet. There are no real benefits to consuming candy, or other processed sweets. Low carb dieters should avoid these foods as they only provide empty calories from processed carb sources. There are much better choices for simple sugars if desired.

Pastries and Desserts: Cakes, cookies, muffins, and other baked goods are typically high in carbs, & also unhealthy fats. These foods provide high calories, with little to no nutritional value.

Soda: Typical soda is high in sugar and should be replaced with water, herbal tea, or other low carb beverages. Diet soda may not contain the carbs of a regular soda pop, but limiting them or avoiding them all together is still ideal for someone on a low carb diet.

Fruit Juice: Even 100% fruit juice contains a lot of sugar and carbs. Someone on a low carb diet may want to limit their fruit juice intake. Fruit juice is a better choice than soda, or other soft drinks. But a low carb dieter should still be mindful of the carbs that come with a glass of fruit juice.

High Carb Vegetables

Potatoes: Including sweet potatoes, while providing nutritional value in other aspects, they are high in carbs and should be limited by low carb dieters.

Corn: High in carbs, and provide little nutritional value. Corn should be avoided on a low carb diet.

Peas: Although nutritious, peas are higher in carbs compared to other vegetables. They should be limited in a low carb diet.

Butternut Squash: Higher in carbs than many other vegetables, but can be enjoyed in small amounts. Not everyone needs to avoid such vegetables completely. Just be mindful of the carbohydrate value in them.

Legumes

Beans: Including black beans, kidney beans, and lentils, are all high in carbs. While providing an excellent source of nutrition, beans often need to be limited, or avoided by a low carb dieter.

Fruits

Bananas: High in carbs and natural sugars, should be limited or avoided. Not everyone needs to completely avoid banana's as they have nutritional value. Be aware of the carbs they come with & enjoy if they fit into your diet plan.

Grapes: Higher in carbs and sugars than most fruits, grapes should be eaten sparingly.

Mangoes: Contain a lot of sugar and carbs. Limit them according to your personal diet plan.

Pineapple: Another high sugar, high carb fruit to limit or avoid on a low carb diet.

Processed Foods

Snack Foods: Chips, crackers, and other processed snack foods are usually high in carbs and unhealthy fats. That's is not a good combination for low carb dieters.

Frozen Meals: Many frozen meals contain hidden carbs and sugars. It is always best to get nutrition from whole food sources. Limit these types of foods, or avoid them all together.

Fast Food: Often high in carbs due to breading, sauces, and sides like fries. When eating out, ask for the low carb options.

Alcoholic Beverages

Beer: High in sugars & carbs, beer should be limited or avoided.

Sweet Wines and Cocktails: Contain added sugars and are high in carbs. Stick to dry wines or spirits mixed with low carb mixers, or avoid completely.

By limiting or avoiding these high carb foods, you can better manage your carb intake and stay on track with your low carb diet. Opting for healthier, low carb alternatives can make it easier to adhere to your dietary goals while still enjoying a variety of delicious foods.

Importance of Meal Planning

Meal planning is a crucial aspect of maintaining a low carb diet. It helps ensure you have the right ingredients on hand, makes grocery shopping more efficient, and reduces the temptation to stray from your dietary goals. By planning your meals in advance, you can maintain a balanced diet, save time, and make healthier choices.

Tips for Effective Meal Planning

Plan Ahead: Set aside time each week to plan your meals. Choose recipes that are simple to prepare and align with your dietary preferences.

Batch Cooking: Prepare large portions of meals and store them as individual servings. This makes it easy to grab a healthy, low carb meal on busy days.

Variety: Incorporate a variety of foods to keep your meals interesting and nutritious. Rotate different proteins, vegetables, and healthy fats.

Use a Shopping List: Write down all the ingredients you need for the week. This helps avoid impulse purchases and ensures you have everything required for your recipes.

Prep Ingredients: Chop vegetables, marinate meats, and prepare sauces ahead of time. This reduces cooking time during the week and makes meal preparation easier.

Managing Sugar Cravings

Cravings for high-carb foods can be one of the most challenging aspects of maintaining a low-carb diet. These cravings can be triggered by various factors, including stress, boredom, or nutritional deficiencies. Understanding the root cause of your cravings can help you manage them more effectively.

Tips to Manage Cravings

Stay Hydrated: Sometimes, thirst is mistaken for hunger. Drinking water regularly can help reduce cravings.

Eat Regularly: Skipping meals can lead to intense hunger and cravings, which can cause binge eating. Aim to eat balanced meals and snacks at regular intervals.

Include Healthy Fats and Proteins: These macronutrients can help you feel full and satisfied, reducing the urge to snack on high-carb foods.

Get Enough Sleep: Lack of (quality of) sleep can disrupt hunger hormones and increase cravings.

Stay Busy: Engaging in activities or hobbies can distract you from cravings and reduce the likelihood of mindless eating.

Enjoying Higher Carb Foods Occasionally

While maintaining a low-carb diet, one may wish to enjoy their favorite higher-carb foods occasionally. This can help prevent feelings of deprivation and promote long-term adherence to your dietary plan.

Strategy Tips for Enjoying High Carb Foods

Plan Ahead: Schedule your higher-carb meals or treats in advance. This allows you to balance them within your overall diet.

Portion Control: Enjoy smaller portions of your favorite high-carb foods to satisfy your cravings without overindulging.

Balance Your Meal: Combine higher-carb foods with proteins and healthy fats to slow down the absorption of carbohydrates and maintain stable blood sugar levels.

Choose Quality Carbs: Opt for high-quality, nutrient-dense carb sources like whole grains, fruits, and vegetables instead of processed foods.

Mindful Eating: Eat slowly and savor each bite. Mindful eating can enhance your enjoyment and prevent overeating.

Managing cravings and incorporating occasional higher-carb foods can make a low-carb diet more sustainable and enjoyable. By planning ahead, practicing portion control, and choosing high-quality carb sources, you can indulge in your favorite treats without derailing your dietary goals.

Tips for Dining Out on a Low-Carb Diet

Research the Restaurant Menu:
Before heading out, take a few minutes to review the restaurant's menu online if possible. Many restaurants provide detailed descriptions of their dishes, including nutritional information online on their websites. This can help you identify low-carb options and make informed choices.

Ask for Modifications:
Don't hesitate to ask for modifications to make your meal more low-carb friendly. Most restaurants are accommodating and can tailor dishes to meet your dietary needs. Common modifications include:
Substitute starchy sides: Request vegetables, salad, or a side of avocado instead of fries, rice, or bread.
Hold the bread: Ask for sandwiches or burgers without the bun, or replace it with lettuce wraps.
-Skip the sauce: Many sauces and dressings are high in sugar and carbs. Request them on the side or opt for olive oil and vinegar.

Focus on Protein and Vegetables:
When choosing your meal, prioritize dishes that feature protein and vegetables. Some good options include:
Grilled meats and seafood: Look for grilled chicken, steak, fish, or shrimp.

Salads: Choose salads with a protein source, such as chicken, beef, or fish, and ask for low-carb dressings.
Vegetable sides: Steamed or sautéed vegetables make excellent low-carb sides.

Be Wary of Hidden Carbs:

Many dishes may contain hidden carbs in the form of breading, sauces, or marinades. Ask your server about the ingredients and preparation methods to avoid unexpected carb intake. Key items to watch out for include:
Breading and batter: Opt for grilled or baked instead of fried foods.
Sweet sauces and glazes: Avoid or limit dishes with sugary sauces like teriyaki, barbecue, or sweet chili.
Dressings: Choose oil-based dressings or bring your own low-carb dressing.

Dining out on a low-carb diet is entirely feasible with a bit of planning and communication. By researching the menu, asking for modifications, focusing on protein and vegetables, and being mindful of hidden carbs, you can enjoy eating out without compromising your dietary goals.

Grocery Shopping Tips for Low-Carb Eating

Make a Weekly Meal Plan:
Plan your meals for the week, including breakfasts, lunches, dinners, and snacks. This helps you stay organized and focused on low-carb choices.

Include a variety of proteins, healthy fats, and low-carb vegetables in your plan to ensure balanced nutrition.

Create a Detailed Shopping List:
Based on your meal plan, make a comprehensive shopping list. Organize it by categories such as produce, meats, dairy, and pantry items.

Stick to your list to avoid impulse buys that may not fit into your low-carb diet.

Check Labels and Ingredients:
Read nutrition labels carefully to check for hidden sugars and high-carb ingredients.

Avoid products with added sugars, high-fructose corn syrup, and refined grains.

Shopping Strategies

Shop the Perimeter:
Focus on the outer aisles of the grocery store where fresh produce, meats, dairy, and eggs are typically located.

Limit time spent in the inner aisles, which often contain processed and high-carb foods.

Stock Up on Low-Carb Staples:

Keep a variety of low-carb staples on hand, such as eggs, leafy greens, cruciferous vegetables, avocados, nuts, seeds, and cheese.

Choose lean meats, fish, and poultry, as well as healthy fats like olive oil, coconut oil, and butter.

Buy in Bulk When Possible:

Purchase non-perishable low-carb items in bulk to save money and ensure you have them on hand.

Look for Fresh and Seasonal Produce:

Choose fresh, seasonal vegetables to get the best flavor and nutritional value.

Experiment with a variety of low-carb vegetables to keep your meals interesting.

Budget-Friendly Tips

Use Coupons and Discounts:
Look for coupons and discounts on low-carb products and produce. Many stores offer digital coupons that can be loaded onto your loyalty card.

Sign up for store newsletters and apps to receive notifications about sales and special offers.

Consider Frozen and Canned Options:
Frozen vegetables can be a convenient and budget-friendly option, especially when fresh produce is out of season.

Choose canned vegetables and meats with no added sugars or preservatives. Rinse canned vegetables to reduce sodium content if desired.

Avoid Processed Low-Carb Products:
Many processed low-carb products can be expensive and may contain questionable ingredients.

Focus on whole, unprocessed foods for the majority of your diet to save money and improve overall health.

By following these grocery shopping tips, you can make informed choices that support your low-carb lifestyle while managing your budget effectively.

Easy 7 Day Sample Low-Carb Meal Plans

Day 1

Breakfast:
- Scrambled eggs with spinach and feta cheese
- Half an avocado
- Black coffee or herbal tea

Lunch:
- Grilled chicken salad with mixed greens, cherry tomatoes, cucumber, and olive oil dressing
- A handful of almonds

Dinner:
- Baked salmon with lemon and dill
- Steamed broccoli and cauliflower with butter
- Mixed green side salad with vinaigrette

Snack:
- Greek yogurt with a few raspberries and a sprinkle of chia seeds

Day 2

Breakfast:
- Omelette with mushrooms, bell peppers, and cheese
- A small handful of berries
- Green tea

Lunch:
- Lettuce wraps with turkey, avocado, bacon, and tomato
- Sliced cucumber with hummus

Dinner:
- Beef stir-fry with broccoli, bell peppers, and zucchini, cooked in coconut oil
- Cauliflower rice

Snack:
- Celery sticks with almond butter

Day 3

Breakfast:
- Chia seed pudding made with unsweetened almond milk, topped with a few nuts and seeds
- Black coffee

Lunch:
- Tuna salad with mixed greens, olives, cherry tomatoes, and a boiled egg
- A small portion of cheese

Dinner:
- Roast chicken thighs with rosemary and garlic
- Sautéed green beans with butter
- Mixed green salad with olive oil and lemon dressing

Snack:
- A small portion of mixed nuts

Day 4

Breakfast:
- Smoothie made with spinach, avocado, unsweetened almond milk, and a scoop of protein powder
- Herbal tea

Lunch:
- Grilled shrimp with a side of asparagus and mixed greens
- A small handful of macadamia nuts

Dinner:
- Pork chops with a creamy mustard sauce
- Roasted Brussels sprouts
- Cauliflower mash

Snack:
- Cottage cheese with a few sliced strawberries

Day 5

Breakfast:
- Boiled eggs with a side of sautéed kale
- A few slices of smoked salmon
- Black coffee

Lunch:
- Chicken Caesar salad with homemade dressing (no croutons)
- A few cherry tomatoes

Dinner:
- Zucchini noodles with marinara sauce and meatballs
- Side salad with mixed greens, cucumber, and olive oil dressing

Snack:
- Bell pepper strips with guacamole

Day 6

Breakfast:
- Bacon and eggs with a side of sautéed mushrooms
- Green tea

Lunch:
- Turkey and cheese roll-ups with a side of baby carrots
- A small handful of pecans

Dinner:
- Grilled steak with garlic butter
- Steamed asparagus
- Mixed green salad with avocado and olive oil dressing

Snack:
- A few slices of cheese with olives

Day 7

Breakfast:
- Almond flour pancakes with a small amount of sugar-free syrup
- Black coffee

Lunch:
- Spinach and feta stuffed chicken breast
- Cucumber and tomato salad with balsamic vinegar

Dinner:
- Lamb chops with mint sauce
- Roasted cauliflower with parmesan cheese
- Mixed green salad with lemon vinaigrette

Snack:
- Greek yogurt with a few blueberries and a sprinkle of flaxseeds

These simple sample meal plans provide a variety of delicious and satisfying low-carb options, ensuring you get a balance of nutrients while keeping your carbohydrate intake low. Adjust portion sizes and ingredients as needed to fit your dietary preferences and nutritional requirements.

List of 50 Fruits With Approximate Carbohydrate Content per 100 grams/3.5 oz/1/2 Cup:

1. *Apple: 14.0 g*
2. *Banana: 22.8 g*
3. *Orange: 11.8 g*
4. *Grapes: 18.1 g*
5. *Strawberries: 7.7 g*
6. *Blueberries: 14.5 g*
7. *Watermelon: 7.6 g*
8. *Pineapple: 13.1 g*
9. *Mango: 14.8 g*
10. *Kiwi: 15.1 g*
11. *Peach: 9.5 g*
12. *Pear: 15.5 g*
13. *Plum: 9.9 g*
14. *Apricot: 11.1 g*
15. *Cherry: 16.0 g*
16. *Raspberry: 11.9 g*
17. *Blackberry: 9.6 g*

18. Cranberry: 12.2 g
19. Papaya: 10.8 g
20. Guava: 14.3 g
21. Passion fruit: 23.4 g
22. Lemon: 9.3 g
23. Lime: 10.5 g
24. Grapefruit: 9.2 g
25. Avocado: 8.5 g
26. Fig: 16.3 g
27. Pomegranate: 18.7 g
28. Persimmon: 18.6 g
29. Date: 74.0 g
30. Lychee: 16.5 g
31. Tangerine: 13.3 g
32. Nectarine: 11.3 g
33. Cantaloupe: 8.2 g
34. Honeydew melon: 9.1 g
35. Coconut (fresh): 15.2 g
36. Star fruit (Carambola): 3.9 g
37. Jackfruit: 23.3 g
38. Kiwano (Horned melon): 5.3 g
39. Ackee: 14.0 g
40. Plantain: 31.9 g
41. Breadfruit: 27.1 g

42. *Cherimoya: 16.3 g*
43. *Longan: 15.1 g*
44. *Buddha's hand: 14.0 g*
45. *Ugli fruit: 8.4 g*
46. *Feijoa: 12.9 g*
47. *Quince: 15.3 g*
48. *Jujube: 18.0 g*
49. *Persimmon (Japanese): 18.6 g*
50. *Loganberry: 10.2 g*

Please note that carbohydrate content can vary slightly depending on factors such as ripeness and variety. These values are approximate and sourced from various nutritional databases.

List of 50 Vegetables Along with Approximate Carbohydrate Content Per 100 grams/3.5 oz/1/2 Cup:

1. Spinach: 3.6 g
2. Broccoli: 6.6 g
3. Carrots: 9.6 g
4. Tomatoes: 3.9 g
5. Cabbage: 5.8 g
6. Bell peppers (green): 4.6 g
7. Bell peppers (red): 6.0 g
8. Onions: 9.3 g
9. Lettuce (Romaine): 3.3 g
10. Cauliflower: 4.9 g
11. Zucchini: 3.1 g
12. Eggplant: 5.9 g
13. Cucumber: 3.6 g
14. Green beans: 6.9 g

15. Peas: 14.5 g

16. Asparagus: 3.9 g

17. Brussels sprouts: 8.0 g

18. Kale: 8.7 g

19. Celery: 2.97 g

20. Radishes: 3.4 g

21. Pumpkin: 6.5 g

22. Sweet potato: 20.1 g

23. Potato (white): 17.5 g

24. Potato (sweet): 20.7 g

25. Artichoke: 10.5 g

26. Beets: 9.6 g

27. Turnips: 6.4 g

28. Squash (butternut): 11.7 g

29. Squash (acorn): 9.0 g

30. Mushrooms: 3.3 g

31. Kohlrabi: 6.2 g

32. Rutabaga: 8.6 g

33. Fennel: 7.3 g

34. Bok choy (pak choi): 2.2 g

35. Swiss chard: 3.7 g

36. Watercress: 1.3 g

37. Collard greens: 5.4 g

38. Mustard greens: 4.7 g

39. *Okra: 7.5 g*
40. *Peppers (jalapeño): 4.1 g*
41. *Peppers (banana): 7.0 g*
42. *Peppers (chili): 9.5 g*
43. *Leeks: 14.2 g*
44. *Garlic: 29.0 g*
45. *Ginger: 17.8 g*
46. *Bean sprouts: 3.9 g*
47. *Snow peas: 7.6 g*
48. *Daikon radish: 4.1 g*
49. *Chayote: 3.6 g*
50. *Parsnips: 17.0 g*

Please note that carbohydrate content can vary slightly depending on factors such as cooking method and variety. These values are approximate and sourced from various nutritional databases.

List of 10 Dairy Options Low in Carbs, With Carbohydrate Content Per 100 grams/3.5 oz/1/2 Cups:

1. Cream Cheese: 3.4 g
2. Feta Cheese: 4.1 g
3. Cottage Cheese: 3.4 g
4. Mozzarella Cheese: 2.2 g
5. Parmesan Cheese: 3.2 g
6. Greek Yogurt (plain): 3.6 g
7. Ricotta Cheese: 3.4 g
8. Brie Cheese: 0.5 g
9. Camembert Cheese: 0.4 g
10. Swiss Cheese: 0.4 g

These values can vary slightly depending on the brand and specific type of product. Always check the nutrition label for the most accurate information.

List of 30 High-Carb Foods with Approximate Carbohydrate Content per 100 grams/3.5 oz/1/2 Cups:

1. *White Bread: 49 g*
2. *Bagels: 50 g*
3. *Pasta (cooked): 25 g*
4. *Rice (white, cooked): 28 g*
5. *Potatoes (white, boiled): 17 g*
6. *Potato Chips: 54 g*
7. *French Fries: 37 g*
8. *Cereal (sweetened): 47 g*
9. *Granola: 64 g*
10. *Pizza (regular crust): 30 g*
11. *Cookies: 55 g*
12. *Cake: 46 g*
13. *Muffins: 50 g*
14. *Donuts: 50 g*
15. *Ice Cream (regular): 21 g*

16. *Chocolate (milk chocolate): 40 g*
17. *Honey: 62 g*
18. *Maple Syrup: 67 g*
19. *Jam: 51 g*
20. *Raisins: 79 g*
21. *Dates: 75 g*
22. *Corn (sweet, cooked): 19 g*
23. *Peas (cooked): 14 g*
24. *Sweet Potatoes (boiled): 17 g*
25. *Plantains (fried): 31 g*
26. *Quinoa (cooked): 21 g*
27. *Buckwheat (cooked): 18 g*
28. *Millet (cooked): 23 g*
29. *Barley (cooked): 28 g*
30. *Couscous (cooked): 24 g*

These values are approximate and can vary based on cooking methods and specific brands. It's important to check nutrition labels for accurate carbohydrate content when selecting foods for a low-carb diet.

Balancing daily life while adhering to a low-carb diet requires thoughtful planning and commitment to healthy choices. By prioritizing nutrient-dense foods such as lean proteins, non-starchy vegetables, and healthy fats, individuals can maintain stable energy levels throughout the day. It's essential to incorporate variety and creativity into meals to prevent monotony and ensure satisfaction. Additionally, practicing mindful eating and being aware of carb content in foods can help in making informed dietary decisions. Ultimately, striking a balance between enjoying food and achieving health goals involves understanding personal preferences, making sustainable choices, and embracing a lifestyle that supports both physical well-being and overall satisfaction.

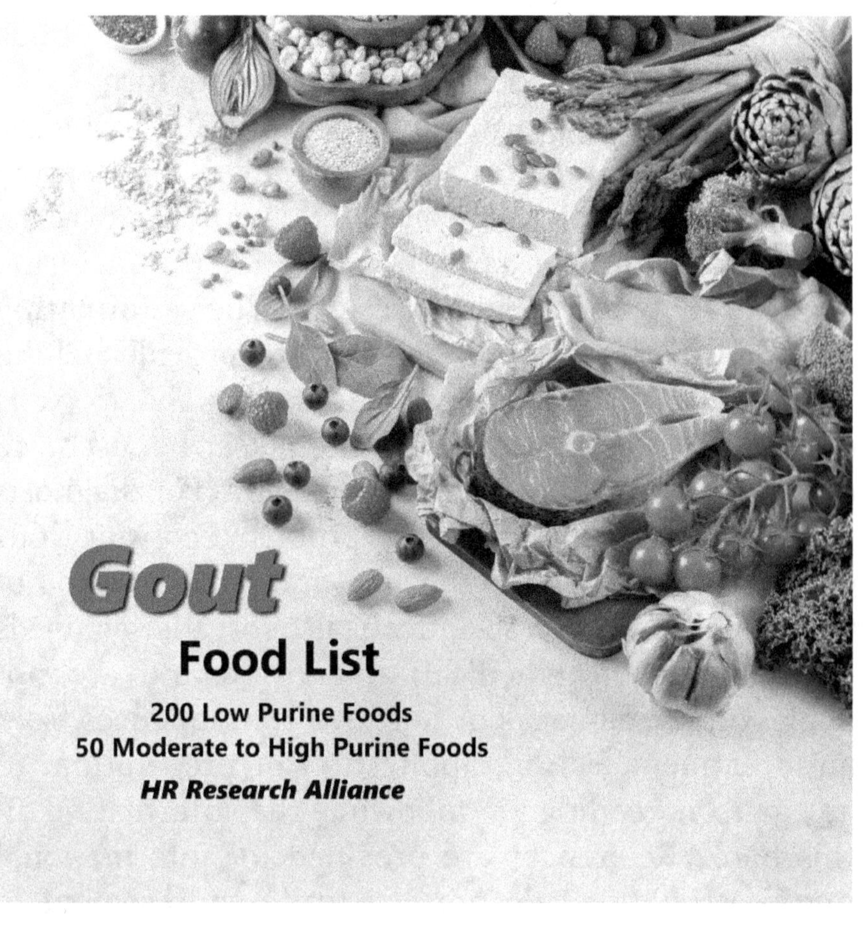

More food content lists.